CANCER
Understanding Cancer, Prevention & Reversal with a Plant Based Diet

The Medicine On Your Plate – Vol 3

By John Hodges & Ted Gif

www.viddapublishing.com

This edition published by
VIDDA Publishing Ltd in 2015. www.viddapublishing.com
Copyright © VIDDA Publishing Ltd 2015

While the author has made all reasonable efforts to ensure that the information contained in this book is accurate and up to date at the time of publication, anyone reading this book should note the following important points:-

Medical and pharmaceutical knowledge are constantly changing and the author and the publisher cannot and do not guarantee the accuracy or appropriateness of the contents of this book;

In any event, this book is not intended to be, and should not be relied upon, as a substitute for appropriate, tailored professional advice. Both the author and the publisher strongly recommend that a doctor or other healthcare professional is consulted before embarking on major dietary changes;

For the reasons set out above, and to the fullest extent permitted by law, the author and publisher: (i) cannot and do not accept any legal duty of care or responsibility in relation to the accuracy or appropriateness of the contents of this book, even where expressed as 'advice' or using other words to this effect; and (ii) disclaim any liability, loss, damage or risk that may be claimed or incurred as a consequence - directly or indirectly - of the use and/or application of any of the contents of this book.

Cover design by John Hodges.

VIDDA Publishing BOOK SHELF:
www.viddapublishing.com/books.html

Have you thought about self-publishing via Amazon Kindle? If so to make the process easier and more productive, I highly recommend this software to help you on your way.

KBookPromotion: bit.ly/KBookPromotion

Your FREE Gift

Thank you for purchasing this book. To show our appreciation we would like to offer you a copy of our FREE recipe book "BRING LIFE TO YOUR FOOD". To download, visit our website: **www.viddapublishing.com**.

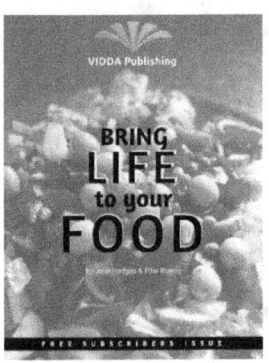

If you're interested in Health, Nutrition, Green and / or Cruelty-Free products please visit our Websites and online **VIDDA Health Stores** (US: bit.ly/VIDDAstore & UK: bit.ly/VIDDAstoreUK).

www.viddapublishing.com

www.sirtfood.com

www.themedicineonyourplate.com

www.greenupyourlife.org

www.ecologizatuvida.com

Table of Content

Introduction

In a book of approximately 14,000 words, it is almost impossible to describe in any detail the enormity of the condition we refer to as cancer. This text, then, will explain in general terms what is meant by the term cancer and the entirely natural biological processes involved in its genesis. The reader will be introduced to some key scientific terms which are central to our understanding of the collective of diseases we refer to as cancer. After such knowledge has been imparted the reader will gain an appreciation of the role of diet in cancer prevention. It is well beyond the remit of this writing to discuss the role of diet in terms of a cure for cancer and the discussion should not impart that following a balanced diet is a substitute for a prescribed therapy. I do not doubt the testimonials of cancer suffers that I came across in the course of the research for this book. However, there is a clear difference between notions of *"prevention"* and notions of *"cure"*, they are, to put it bluntly, entirely different propositions. The text will provide empirical evidence concerning the activity of various biological molecules and nutrients which could well in time be proven to express cancer prevention properties. In my view, as research continues such an eventuality is only a matter of time. As an opposite proposition, the penultimate chapter will provide examples of specific chemicals that have been shown to be implicated in specific cancers. I see no reason why in time it will not be established that substance Z will destroy the tumours associated with Cancer A and that foodstuff B is a source of such a substance. The substances which we consume as a part of the balanced diet should be eaten as a matter, of course, irrespective of any cancer-fighting abilities. The reader will hopefully appreciate why cancer is such a difficult set of diseases to defeat. This book is a call to all of us to exercise our own power and initiate the necessary dietary changes which have been shown to improve the metabolism. As such it may be helpful for the reader to view the assertions contained herein as sound biological reasons to think about what we are eating. Finally, the reader should appreciate that the advice contained herein is not a set of rules or commandments they are suggestions based on empirical scientific evidence and as such the reader is invited to comment, question, enquire or otherwise interact with the suppositions presented below. With reference to specific examples, the final chapter will provide an indication of the market-driven nature of cancer treatment.

Chapter 1:
What is Cancer?

Along with serious health conditions such as Heart Disease, HIV, Ebola, Alzheimer's disease or an inherited disorder such as Huntington's disease, a cancer diagnosis is going to change your life and the lives of those around you forever. A diagnosis of such diseases is supremely likely to elicit a whirlwind of emotional responses of stratospheric proportions. When we hear the word *"cancer"* we automatically become frightened and there is no point in sugar coating this fact or pretending that cancer is somehow not a serious and life-threatening condition. To put it into perspective, according to the charity Cancer Research UK (CRUK), half of the UK population born after 1960 will develop some form of cancer. If CRUK is correct half of the UK population that are approaching or have just passed their half century, will get a cancer diagnosis. This is in part due to the demographics of the UK, which is home to an ageing population and it is important to state that cancer is primarily a disease symptomatic of old age. According to Dr Peter Sasieni, the leader of the team who carried out the research, over 60% of all cancers are diagnosed in people aged over 65.

As of 2011, in the UK approximately 250,000 new diagnoses of cancer are recorded annually and roughly 130,000 die from the disease. This mortality occurs against a backdrop in which almost two million people are living with one form of cancer or another. However, the good news is that cancer is not the death sentence it used to be. Overall, survival rates are improving and for the UK it was reported in early 2014 that for the first time the number of people surviving the disease has surpassed those who have died, which is clearly fantastic news. Having said that the UK survival rates are significantly lower than those for other European countries, which as this hyperlink (http://bit.ly/1xYWsNc) makes abundantly clear is as shocking as it is unnecessary. Speaking personally, I have no idea how I would react to a diagnosis, but I do know I'd need plenty of love and support from my nearest and dearest. Cancer is a disease which is not bound by human constructs and it is certainly not constrained by age, gender or ethnicity and we are reminded of this fact on a regular basis. For instance, the unexpected death of the supreme writing talent that was Iain Banks was an unpleasant surprise, to say the least. According to the deceased, he was diagnosed with cancer of the gall bladder in the spring of 2013, by June of the same year, aged 59 the author died at home with his family. Prior to his death, he is reported to have asked his long-term partner Adele Hartley if she would "*do me the honour of becoming my widow*". If you can't appreciate this kind of gallows humour and you have not read any of his books, I urge you to remedy that particular situation as soon as you are able.

The global statistics are sobering and in a real sense is the stuff of nightmares. In 2008 approximately thirteen million new cancer cases were diagnosed and 8 million individuals were killed by the collective of diseases which fall under the umbrella term cancer. The latest press release from the World Health Organisation (WHO) asserts that death rates are steadily rising. Figures from this international institution state clearly and plainly that cancer is still a leading cause of death, such that in 2012, about 14 million new cases were diagnosed and over 8 million individuals still die annually as a result of their condition. Without a doubt, a portion of these figures can be attributed to the fact that we are living longer and as we age the chances of us developing cancer progressively increases. It is also true that the usual and established suspects of smoking, excessive alcohol consumption, exposure to synthetic chemicals, obesity (unhealthy eating habits) and a lack of regular exercise are the principle drivers for the upward trend in the cancer figures.

The figures themselves mask a crucial point, which is that the medical profession does not consider cancer a single disease. There are in fact over 100 different types of cancer and therefore each requires a unique and personal treatment regimen. For men, by far the biggest killer is cancer of the lungs rapidly followed by prostate, colorectal, stomach and liver cancer. For women, the biggest killers are breast, colorectal, lung, cervix and stomach cancer. The reader should be assured that cancer is a slow, degenerative and in its later stages excruciatingly painful disease. Suffice it to say, that given a choice cancer would be well toward the bottom of my options for leaving this mortal coil. Overall, the mortality rates are depending on the cancer in question up to 20% higher for men than they are for women. Sorry guys (including yours truly) but *"them's the shakes"*. As of 2013, it is estimated that over half of all new diagnoses and almost two-thirds of all deaths occur in the majority world (the Global South). The prognosis from the WHO is that by 2030 twenty-two million new cases of cancer per year will be diagnosed and 13 million people per year will die from the disease, with roughly 70% of this figure being in the global south (Asia, Africa and Latin America). These figures are cumulative and so do not represent the total diagnoses or deaths, and as such cancer is doubtless one of our most potent killers. Having said that the survival rate around the world is steadily improving, subject to variables such as:

- Cancer in question.

- Stage of progression when the diagnosis was made.

- Lifestyle and dietary factors.

- Genetic and hereditary (family history) factors.

All of this has I hope to set the scene for the last section of this chapter which is to ask succinctly *"what is cancer?"*

The human body is in effect the most highly evolved and complex molecular machine on planet Earth. It is a biological machine composed almost entirely of trillions of living cells which collectively divide and reproduce billions of times every day. Aside from the gametes (which reproduce sexually by meiosis) all the cells which reproduce in the human body, do so by mitosis. In biology, the cells of the body are often referred to as somatic cells and the way they divide (mitosis) is often called asexual reproduction. In asexual reproduction, the two *"daughter"* cells have exactly the same number of chromosomes as the *"parent"* cell. Hence the daughter and parent cells are identical, which if you think about it makes perfect sense! The process of mitosis is itself highly complex and continuous process and different cell types reproduce at different rates. Mitosis itself takes between 30 and 90 minutes depending on the biological structure in question. A principle reason for cell division is that cells do not live forever and so must be replaced by new identical cells. Hence, one facet of the complexity of the communication which exists between cells is the rate at which they undergo mitosis. The essential point about cancer is that it starts from one mutated cell whose characteristics are passed on to all daughter cells. To explain this we must impart what is meant by the term mutation and this means we must refer to the structure of Deoxyribonucleic Acid (DNA). The contentious discovery of the structure of DNA in 1953 is officially credited to James Watson and Francis Crick. However, the story is not that simple and like all critical scientific discoveries, the story is a pot boiler of epically nefarious proportions which could (arguably) raise even the eyebrows of the fictional character "the Prince" as penned by Niccolo Machiavelli. If the reader wishes to find out more then follow this link (http://bit.ly/1d7SZQP) and begin your journey into classic scientific intrigue double cross and even plain theft, and then you decide!

The DNA molecule is held together by structures known as organic bases, which only the only bond together such that thymine (T) bonds only to adenine (A) or vice versa, or guanine (G) bonds only to cytosine (C) or vice versa. If this does not occur such that the sequence of base pairs changes then a mutation has occurred. For example, in sickle cell anaemia, the base pair T-A is substituted for an alternative pair C-G, and the result is the characteristic sickle cell as opposed to the normal concave circular shape of the red blood cell. In the *"sickle"* shape the red blood cells are unable to transport oxygen and can clump together (aggregate) making the person more prone to blood clots. On the other hand, in regions where malaria is a fact of daily life the sickle cell shape represents a trade-off because the *plasmodium falciparum* and *plasmodium vivax* parasites which cause malaria cannot complete their life cycle if there are too many sickle cells. When the DNA molecule is changed in this manner, it is said to be mutated and a substance which causes mutation is termed a mutagen. Concurrently, as cancer is caused by the mutation of a single cell a mutagen which causes cancer is termed a carcinogen and the process of cancer initiation is known as carcinogenesis. Mutation is a common feature of biology and occurs due to alterations in the base pairing structure of DNA. Put simply, DNA and protein synthesis is a complex biochemical process and mistakes happen. Normally mutations result in cells that cannot perform life processes themselves, which results in cell apoptosis or cell suicide.

Alternatively, the mutated cells are detected and destroyed by the immune system. In the case of cancer, neither of these essential processes occurs and so cancer cells begin accumulating at the site of carcinogenesis. If the reader wishes to explore in more detail the terms explained in this paragraph please feel free to peruse this hyperlink: *http://bit.ly/1WZjFfV.*

Cancer is characterised by repeated and unregulated cell division, the result is a mass of cells known as a tumour. As a general rule, once a tumour is detected it can contain as many as a billion cancerous cells. The tumour itself can be *"benign"* or *"malignant",* but the designation is not absolute because it is possible for the tumour to vacillate between the two states. At its absolute simplest a benign tumour does not spread whilst a malignant tumour will. Cancer which has spread and caused a secondary tumour is said to have undergone metastasis. Unfortunately, most cancers have the capacity to shed cells and once this occurs the person concerned really is in trouble as up to 90% of all cancer fatalities are the result of secondary tumours. All tumours are supplied with nutrients via the lymphatic system and the bloodstream, which together are referred to as the *"circulatory system".* When metastasis occurs, the initial tumour sheds cancerous cells which are then transported via the circulatory system to another location (i.e. organ) within the body and a secondary tumour starts to grow. It can take many months or even years for particular cancer to express itself in the body, let alone be detected, on the other hand as with Iain Banks cancer may kill you in a matter of weeks. In other words, although lung and breast cancer kills more people, cancer such as of the prostate gland or the gall bladder can prove to be fatal much more rapidly. In cancerous cells, the biological processes which regulate and control mitosis are circumvented. The cancerous cells simply do not receive the chemical instruction to stop dividing and cellular death (or apoptosis) does not occur. Cancerous cells (which are exact copies of the parent cell) are larger, divide uncontrollably and more rapidly than healthy cells and as they do so utilise more of the nutrients that would be used in healthy metabolism. So *"a cancer"* can loosely be stated as a situation in which one abnormal cell starts to divide by mitosis and then its daughter cells continue the process abnormally. For example, in a condition known as hairy cell leukaemia (HCL), the affected white blood cells have minuscule hair like structures projecting from the cell membrane. HCL itself is a relatively rare condition but its presence does suppress the production of healthy red and white blood cells in preference to the mutated hairy form. Amongst other consequences the person affected is much more susceptible to secondary infections that may not affect another individual.

Thus, cancer is caused by a genetic mutation which induces carcinogenesis and the mistake can take years to express itself or it may take a few months. This reality is one reason why cancer is not seen as a single disease. Irrespective of the carcinogen involved, once the genes that control cell division have been altered they are termed oncogenes. The term oncogene is derived from the Greek word for mass, (*onkoss*) and the study of cancer and tumours in their entirety is known as oncology. When a cell is mutated by an oncogene the mutation is not detected by the body and so the tumour begins to establish itself and the disease we term *"cancer"* is the result. For most types of cancer, the onset of the disease is a long-term process in which normal cells undergo several stages before they are instructed by the oncogenes to behave in a cancerous manner. Clearly, cancer is a huge and distressing subject which is impossible to cover in one book and so the rest of this text will be exploring the role of diet in both the prevention and cure of cancer. The importance cannot be understated because in the UK and US alone cancer is responsible for 730,000 deaths every year and all over the world the numbers are rising.

Chapter 2:
Diet and Cancer Prevention

In the 21st century, it should be self-evident that eating a balanced diet is absolutely essential to overall health and well-being. In terms of diet and the incidence of cancer, there is no single superfood or dietary regimen that is going in itself to prevent the incidence of cancer. Having said that it is absolutely possible for all of us to take the necessary steps which allow us to make informed decisions about how a particular food or food group may boost the ability of the body to respond to the carcinogens it may be exposed to. According to CRUK the role of diet in cancer prevention is pivotal; the charity openly states that up to 10% of all cancers can be prevented by adopting healthy eating choices. The organisation goes further and states that up to 5% of all cancers could be prevented by maintaining an optimal BMI. In this context it critically important to reiterate that the onus of responsibility for the pollution and environmental destruction which is rife around the planet is not the fault of "concerned citizens" or "activists". The responsibility (which in my view is criminal) lays with the global military-industrial complex (in its widest possible sense) and until the agencies which compose the complex are brought to trial, said criminality will continue. This chapter will outline how we as individuals can best look after ourselves, which means taking control of the information you believe and wherever possible acting accordingly. For example, if you are concerned about the destruction of mangrove forest in South East Asia to make way for prawn and shrimp farming, (amongst other activities) then don't buy prawns from that part of the world. According to research published in the journal Bioscience," some 35% of all mangrove forest has been lost since the 1990's. Hence, following on from the *"meat is murder"* argument mentioned in *"crushing diabetes"*, one could stop eating farmed crustaceans altogether and actively consider the virtues of a plant based diet instead.

Thus, this chapter will consider the practical steps that we as individuals can take in terms of our diet to prevent or at least delay the incidence of cancer. Such a task is impossible to fully address in one book, principally due to the sheer numbers of different types of cancer and the different biological mechanisms (most of which we do not fully understand) by which they impact on the body. It is perhaps more realistic to ask whether *"eating a particular food or food group can prevent the onset of a particular form of cancer?"* As will be made repeatedly inculcated throughout this entire series of books, when we are talking about food consumption we mean fresh, unprocessed and ideally locally sourced and if at all possible organic food products. The key word here is *"ideally"*; in the SIRT FOOD book mention was made of food deserts. The supermarket oligarchy is merely the most visible symptoms of the malaise that have intertwined itself into the global food distribution system, but that is another story! So rest assured dear reader there is no preaching here, all I'm saying is do what you can when you can but be aware of the bigger picture.

At this juncture, we are once again able to reiterate the negative impact of the justifiably much maligned western diet. The research literature is replete with epidemiological (specific population) studies which attempt to correlate the incidence of cancer in first generation migrant and second generation migrant populations with the indigenous populations but additionally with the host region populations. To put it bluntly, the task is beyond monumentally complex. A landmark study carried out in 1965 analysed breast cancer rates of Japanese women and their children who had migrated to the US and compared the different populations as described in the previous sentence. In essence, the study asserts that rates of breast cancer were higher in the migrant population than in the other two populations considered. Although this research clearly implicates *"Western lifestyle and diet"* as a key driver of breast cancer in the migrant population, the genealogy of the family tree played an equally important part with increased rates of breast cancer. In other words, a fusion of diet and genetics presents itself, such that the offspring of migrant Japanese women were more likely to develop breast cancer than their indigenous peers. As if social science is not complicated enough the study reported that migrants who came from a rural environment were less likely to develop breast cancer than those who came from urban settings. To really inculcate the complexity of the syndrome we are dealing with other studies lead to opposite conclusions. A similar 10-year study (1993-2003) published in the British Journal of Cancer (BJC) conducted similar research comparing Indian and Pakistani populations with indigenous British populations. This South Asian cohort is still by far the largest single component of the UK population which considers itself non-white. As with the 1965 study the host population has lower cancer rates as compared to the UK, but the numbers are rising. In addition, research is revealing that the cancer rates across the board for this population are increasing across the UK. Across the board, the BJC study found that for both genders mortality rates were higher in first generation migrants than in subsequent populations.

So, what is the role of diet in all of this? The first point to make clear is that a good and well-balanced diet is by itself not going to cure cancer. Having said that (and once you decide to stop smoking) unhealthy eating habits and a sedentary lifestyle are the two single biggest factors that increase the risk of developing cancer. In terms of diet the figures are staggering; according to researchers at Cardiff University, approximately 600,000 people die every single year from colorectal cancer. Of the approximate 600,000 deaths from cancer which occur annually in the US, about half are diet and lifestyle related. If this is not a call to engage in more exercise and change your eating habits and at least actively consider a plant based diet, then I don't know what is! As this series of books will continually inculcate when the body is overweight or obese the body is metabolically unbalanced. This is obviously undesirable and aside from medical or psychological reasons largely avoidable. In addition overweight and obese people have a greater risk of developing diseases that can kill, which includes cancer. All variables being equal, obese people are more likely to develop a whole host of cancers as compared to their non-obese counterparts. Chapter 3 of the SIRT FOOD book indicates how a person's BMI is calculated. In essence, a good strategy is to limit your portion sizes and eat only when you are actually hungry as well as keeping a food diary. You should also gravitate toward healthy eating choices and avoid those foods which constitute the Western diet. If you are also carrying out some form of physical activity your endocrine (hormonal) and immune system will benefit. Hence you now have two immediately accessible cancer risk reduction factors at your disposal. The links between bad diet, cancer, type-2 diabetes and other undesirable conditions are clear and apparent.

The WHO has stated that up to a third of all cancers in the western world add up to a fifth of those in the majority world are diet related. In other words, if you follow the healthy eating advice which permeates through this whole series of books you have a reduced risk of developing cancer. The next step is to clearly state that people in Europe who follow a plant based diet are up to 40% less likely to develop any form cancer than those who regularly eat meat. The figure will vary between different populations and other factors will influence the degree of cancer incidence, but the essential point remains. One could write an entire encyclopaedia on this subject, but the basic reasons lie with the nutritional content of meat. For example, the saturated fat content of meat, especially red meat is very high and this stimulates the production of the hormones which are implicated in hormonally based cancers such as breast and prostate cancer. Overall, red meat and processed meats garner the highest degree of risk. None of this should infer that eating meat will definitely kill you, this is all about the assessment of risk and prevention. Generally speaking, the cancers most associated with diet are associated with the organs of the human alimentary canal. The most comprehensive study to date concerning the links between diet, lifestyle and cancer is The European Prospective Investigation into Cancer and Nutrition (EPIC). Over 500,000 European citizens from across the continent are participating in the study which seeks to answer the questions that have been raised over the last several decades.

It is self-evident that fresh fruits, pulses, grains, cereals and vegetables of all types contain all of the nutrients that the body needs. However, the key is of course balance; researchers are a long way from quantifiably establishing causative links between specific nutrients and cancer prevention. Any food scientist will state that in terms of cancer prevention different coloured foodstuffs each contain different nutrients and so balance and varied eating is the way forward. For example one 2008 study found that people who eat a wide range of fruit and vegetables reduced their risk of developing cancer as compared to those who did not. In addition the higher the fibre content of the diet the higher is the degree of resistance to developing bowel (colorectal) cancer. In the UK research suggests that a diet rich in fruits and vegetables could help prevent up to $1/20^{th}$ of all recorded cancers. Put simply these foodstuffs contain many of the vitamins, minerals and the fibre we need for a healthy metabolism. In terms of cancer, it is probably easier to state that we know what not to eat overall and that, of course, is the western diet. Chapter three will discuss the active compounds which form the basis of the above assertions. Once again it is crucially important to stress that the foods indicated below should be consumed as a part of a balanced diet. If a diagnosis of cancer has been presented then the advice of a professional should be sought. In addition, it goes without saying that smoking should be ceased immediately and the consumption of alcohol and caffeine-containing drinks should be severely limited.

Chapter 3:
Food and Cancer Prevention

During my time researching this subject I've met plenty of people who were furious at the lack of state funding for research into both "curing cancer" itself and for support services for those affected by the disease. Speaking personally I find it abhorrent that in the UK as of 2013 only 40% of all research into cancer is provided by the state. In essence, the majority of direct state funding for research is geared toward breast, lung, colorectal and prostate cancer, the remaining 60% comes directly from other sources, namely charitable donations and legacies. One can only wonder at the strides that would be made if but a fraction of the billions of pounds of taxpayers money wasted on criminal endeavours such as Iraq and Afghanistan, were ploughed into cancer research and education. In any discussion of cancer, it is not enough to talk of research and cures, we must also discuss any preventative measure and in the context of this series of books, this means diet. Hence this chapter will focus on the active compounds which are believed to have a role in preventing the onset of different cancers. Where possible I will indicate whether a particular compound has a role in preventing specific cancer.

According to the WHO, approximately one-third of all cancers can be prevented by adopting the same basic strategies that can prevent the onset of type 2 diabetes and other symptoms of metabolic imbalance. As has (I hope) been made abundantly clear throughout this series of books wherever possible, we as individuals should be doing everything we can to prevent the onset of diseases such as diabetes and cancer. Hence, identical arguments can be presented for individuals to make the appropriate choices wherever they can as regards to their diet and level of physical activity. That being said the bigger and the more holistic picture concerning the availability of processed foods and marketing thereof cannot be understated. In addition, it is known that there are literally hundreds if not thousands of synthetic and industrial chemicals circulating throughout the environment which supports all life on Earth. The so-called "cocktail" effect of having hundreds of these chemicals dissolved in our fat cells is the continued subject of fierce scientific debate. The point being that we as individuals should be exercising our personal power in terms of employing the right dietary choices to prevent and manage cancer, but it must never be forgotten that it may not be possible for all people all of the time to exercise these choices. In essence, individual action is all well and good but this is no substitute for coordinated global and state-funded initiatives to really get to grips with crushing cancer. Leaving the larger context aside we can seek to establish whether any dietary advice exists which may prevent or slow the onset of specific cancers?

It has been known for decades that dietary fibre is an essential component of any balanced diet. Since the 1970's there has been a clear association between a high fibre diet and a reduced incidence of colorectal cancer. Such assertions are based on yet more epidemiological studies which show low rates of cancer amongst rural populations in Africa as compared to their western diet consuming counterparts. The reasoning lies with the notion of dietary roughage. In short, fibre facilitates rapid and regular excretion as well as dilution of potential carcinogens in the human digestive tract. The foundation is that any potential toxins will, therefore, have a reduced residency and therefore contact time with the alimentary canal. Such assertions appear to be supported by findings which suggest that populations eating a low fibre diet have a higher incidence of this potentially deadly form of cancer. Additionally, unprocessed fibre is a food source for certain species of bacteria in the digestive system. When the fibre is broken down by the bacteria a substance called butyrate is produced which could suppress the growth of tumours in the lower alimentary canal. Butyrate is a fatty acid which is believed to promote apoptosis in cancer cells in the colon, but not in normal healthy cells. Research has yet to establish a causative link but the one factor that is consistently drawn out is that the fibre must be consumed in situ, that is in its natural state. The role of dietary fibre in cancer prevention is far from clear and has been studied since the mid-1980's. The picture is complex and contentious but appears to indicate that dietary fibre from whole grains and cereals has more cancer-suppressing properties than those from vegetables. It must again be stressed that these properties will only assert themselves if the grains are consumed as part of a balanced diet when the person's metabolism is in balance.

Foodstuffs which are widely considered to have a role in preventing carcinogenesis are readily available and include but are not limited to green and root vegetables, herbs, spices and berries. Many day to day foods are concentrated sources of antioxidants (as discussed in the SIRT FOOD book), substances known as phytochemicals as well as the plethora of essential minerals, vitamins and biological molecules we need for healthy metabolism. Common antioxidants include beta-carotene (found in carrots and other colourful vegetables), lycopene (found in tomatoes) as well as the vitamins C and E. These and other important nutrients are found in cruciferous vegetables as well as fruits and other vegetables with characteristic bright colours. The cruciferous vegetables are some of the most important agricultural crops on the planet and are renowned for being exceptionally good for you, regardless of any cancer suppression properties. For our purposes, the Cruciferae family contain a class of compounds called phytochemicals one group of which are termed glucosinolates.

Overall a phytochemical is any plant-derived compound which has a protective or disease preventing function. There are at least a thousand individual phytochemicals and their precise mode of action is not fully understood. However, it is well known that plants use them to protect themselves and research concerning their efficacy on human beings continue apace. The glucosinolates are phytochemicals which contain sulphur and are the cause of the strong aroma associated with mustard, garlic, horseradish, cabbage and the truly revolting but nutritionally important Brussel sprout. When the glucosinolates are broken down they form metabolites known as indoles and it is these compounds which are thought to garner properties which may help prevent breast, colon and prostate cancer. The indoles are thought to be effective because they:

- May promote cell apoptosis (cell death).

- Have demonstrable anti-inflammatory properties.

- May bind to and inactivate carcinogens.

- Protect against damage to DNA by free radicals (as discussed in the SIRT FOOD book).

- Have proven antiviral and antibacterial effects.

- May inhibit both metastasis and blood vessel formation (angiogenesis) inside growing tumours.

To underline the point that there is no great secret to ingesting food which is not only good for you but also could have a role in preventing cancer one must only consider the allium family of root vegetables. This class of food includes garlic, onions, leeks, chives and the spring onions to which they are attached. Again it is the glucosinolates contained within these foods (not their supplements) that may help the body prevent cancer from taking hold. The red colour of tomatoes comes from the presence of a phytochemical known as lycopene which may have a particular role to play in the prevention of prostate cancer. Lycopene may also have a suppressing role in breast, lung and uterine cancer. Lycopene is thought to improve the function of the immune system by helping it to identify the chemical signals produced by tumorous cells. Furthermore, lycopene is thought to disrupt the communication pathways between cancerous cells thus inhibiting their growth. As a general rule of thumb, the "redder" the food the more lycopene it contains, so step forward watermelon, red chillies and peppers as well as pink grapefruit.

The antioxidant properties of berries are well established and so along with fruits should be eaten fresh and unprocessed as often as possible. In terms of cancer prevention strawberry, raspberry and blackberries appear to garner the deepest impact on cancer cells. In addition, strawberries are a concentrated source of antioxidant vitamins and substances such as ellagic acid. Although present in almost 50 individual foodstuffs the most concentrated sources of ellagic acid are berries, nuts and certain fungi. Overall, ellagic acid is believed to have a role in the processes listed above. However, it is not readily absorbed and so must be consumed as part of a balanced diet. Many of the foods mentioned in this chapter also contain one or more of the 4000 compounds known as flavonoids which are known to produce a whole host of health benefits. These benefits include antioxidant properties as well as improved cell signalling capabilities. Research on the cancer mitigation properties of the flavonoids generally focuses on their ability to suppress the efficacy of enzymes which may damage DNA during carcinogenesis, however, no definite pathway has to date been established. In terms of nutritional benefits, carrots and spinach need no introduction. Both of these foodstuffs have well documented antioxidant properties and the various phytochemicals and flavonoids they contain may have a role in the prevention of cancers of the colon, oesophagus, cervix and stomach. Spinach and other leafy green vegetables are also rich sources of substances such as folate, which is a derivative of folic acid, in other words, it belongs to the B vitamin family. Amongst other functions folate facilitates the effective copying of DNA and where necessary it boosts the efficiency of the enzymes involved in the repair of this absolutely essential molecule.

It would be possible to write a complete book on the role of folic acid, folate and the B vitamins in general in cancer prevention. Accordingly, any internet search will reveal the degree of research on this particular aspect of cancer prevention. Overall, these particular B vitamins are found in varying quantities in many foodstuffs and so obtaining them should not (for most of us) be too difficult. In terms of cancer prevention research focuses on the apparent reduction in the risk of developing cancers of the alimentary canal and associated organs involved in digestion. A further branch of research in this area of cancer prevention has established that there are interactions between nutrients and the genetic code contained within the DNA molecule. The cancer suppression properties of folate and other B vitamins centres on their role in modulating the bonding between the base pairs mentioned in chapter one. Folate also plays an effective part in a process known as DNA methylation which is connected to the complicated process of gene silencing. Put simply, a gene is silenced when the characteristic it codes for is not expressed and in terms of cancer one facet concerns the genetic signal to stop cells dividing. DNA methylation is a pivotal process in ensuring that the expression of a particular gene does not occur. At present we are unclear as to the precise role of folate in gene silencing and what the possible impacts on the cell cycle and carcinogenesis could be. Clearly, one could keep writing ad-infinitum on this subject, such an eventuality is of course not possible and so this chapter draws to a somewhat abrupt close. The reason is simple; in my view, no meal is complete without the appropriate herbs and spices. Hence, the remainder of this chapter will explore some of the cancer prevention properties of the wonderful natural flavourings that transform even the most mundane of meals.

Herbs and spices have been with human beings since at least the beginning of Neolithic time, some 12,000 years ago. This time marked the end of the last great ice age and delimits the period of human development known as the Holocene. The Neolithic period was the last period of the Stone Age and preceded the next epoch of humanities time on planet Earth known as the Bronze Age. The Neolithic period is characterised by the cessation of the hunter-gatherer lifestyle and the concurrent gravitation toward agriculture as well as the manufacture of the tools necessary to carry it out. In short, when we first started growing crops and rearing animals, we began to see the need to both preserve and flavour the food we eat. The ancient Egyptians are known to have used spices to preserve the corpses of the dead they embalmed. Across the ancient world, in general, spices were seen as having connections to specific gods and the rituals developed to worship them. The archaeological record is replete with evidence demonstrating that medicinal qualities of herbs, spices and opiates were not lost on these ancient cultures. It is absolutely true that the story of herbs and spices is inextricably intertwined with the story of the development of human culture, warts and all! Put simply an herb is a plant or part thereof utilised to provide healing properties or flavour food. A spice is any plant based substance that is employed in food cooking or preservation, that adds flavour and/or colour. Spices tend to come in a rich array of colours whilst herbs tend to be green and the utility of each in the kitchen is down to a confluence of the sensitivity of your taste buds and culinary prowess!

In the modern world herbs and spices are of great importance not only for their stated purpose but also because of the expanding corpus of knowledge which sets out the molecular basis for their collective health benefits. A crucial point about herbs and spices is that the quantity eaten does not necessarily relate to any hierarchy of importance. Hence, it is helpful to see both herbs and spices as having attributes which extend well beyond their direct culinary use. A nutrient is loosely defined as any substance that garners some beneficial physiological effect for the organism (heterotroph) which ingests, or in the case of plants (autotrophs) makes it. In terms of therapy and prevention of cancer (and other diseases) the three basic variables considered which establish the validity of a given compound are:

- The susceptibility of the individual.

- The effect or mode of action of the compound.

- The exposure to or concentration of the compound.

Clearly, when viewed through the complex prism of human metabolism the scene is just not that simple. Other variables such as the diet itself, the role of microbes in the gut, genetic and environmental factors, will all need to be evaluated before we can even think about saying that compound X has a role to play in mitigating or curing cancer Y. As with food in general if you are cooking regularly, meaning you are regularly making dishes, you are likely to be eating a whole range of herbs and spices as a matter of course. Therefore, it is likely that any cancer prevention properties will already be manifesting themselves in your diet. Indeed as with the foods discussed in chapter two, to have a role in preventing the onset of cancer herbs and spices must fulfil one or more of the following criteria:

- They suppress the carcinogenesis of known carcinogens.

- They work as antioxidants and / or bind with free radicals.

- They disrupt the action of oncogenes.

- They inhibit division and promote apoptosis of cancerous cells.

- They inhibit microbes and enzymes which promote carcinogenesis.

- They reduce inflammation and boost the effectiveness of the immune system.

The benefits of the hundreds of individual herbs and spices have been documented for thousands of years, so it seems reasonable to suppose that some of them may have particular efficacy in preventing, managing and even curing cancer. In one chapter of a short book, only a general overview can be provided and so the reader is again actively encouraged to follow up on the sources presented at the end of this book.

It has been known for decades that long-term inflammation of somatic (body) tissue is a crucial component of the carcinogenic process. Whether they are malignant or benign, tumours change the immediate (cellular) environment around them. In essence, the tumour promotes its own growth and survival (at the expense of healthy cells) by hijacking the biochemical signals and biological molecules which cells use to communicate with each other. This hi-jacking allows further invasion of the primary site and facilitates metastasis to secondary sites. In addition recent research published via the Massachusetts Institute of Technology (MIT) shows a definite link between inflammation and cancers of the pancreas, liver, colon and oesophagus. In essence, inflammation promotes the activity of free radicals and cells which are dividing in an inflamed environment are much more vulnerable to mutation by carcinogens. Many herbs, spices and other nutritional compounds are known to possess anti-inflammatory properties and this is borne out by laboratory experiments on both animals and human cell cultures.

The table below summarises the above text and gives an overview of the type of foods that we can consume to boost the ability of the body to prevent the development of cancer.

APPENDIX: FOODS WHICH MAY HELP PREVENT CANCER

Foodstuff	Active Ingredients	Possible Cancer Preventative Role
Onion, Garlic and Alliums (bulb	Allicin and other sulphur	Breast, colorectal, skin, oesophagal

shaped vegetables)	containing (organo-sulphur) compounds, Flavonoids, anti-bacterial / viral compounds, Antioxidant compounds, Enzyme boosting compounds, Fibre, Ellagic and similar acids,	and lung cancer, gastrointestinal cancers, induces cell apoptosis
Cruciferae Spinach broccoli, chard, Brussel sprouts et al	Folate, Folic Acid, Antioxidant vitamins, trace minerals, phytochemicals, flavonoids, fibre, indoles	Stomach, mouth and throat cancer, alimentary canal and gastrointestinal cancers, regulate the cell cycle
Tomatoes, carrots, nuts mushrooms, peaches, apples	Lycopene, Beta-carotene (an anti-oxidant), carotenoids trace minerals, Vitamin C and A, lentinan (and other polysaccharides), Anti-tumorigenic	Breast cancer boosts efficacy of immune system, bladder, prostate and testicular cancer, gastrointestinal cancer, breast cancer

Beetroot, red cherries and grapes, purple / dark coloured fruits and vegetables, strawberries, red and yellow peppers	Resveratrol, Anthocyanin and other flavonoids, trace minerals	Colorectal cancer, gastrointestinal cancers, mouth and throat cancer, colorectal cancers, cervical, ovarian and uterine cancer
Herbs Basil, Fennel, Cardamom, Dill, Pepper, most household herbs, apple cider vinegar	Anti-inflammatory, Anti-mutagenic, Anti-tumorigenic, Antiviral, Antibacterial, boost efficacy of DNA repair and detoxifying enzymes, modification of known carcinogenic compounds, linalool (a type of alcohol)	Lung cancer, colorectal cancer, cancers of the alimentary canal (and associated tissues and organs), prostate cancer , mouth and throat cancer, stomach cancer, liver cancer,
Spices Ginger, Turmeric, cinnamon, coriander, cumin, turmeric-mixed	Anti-inflammatory, Anti-mutagenic, Anti-tumorigenic, Antiviral,	Lung cancer, colorectal cancer, cancers of the alimentary canal (and associated tissues and organs),

spices, cloves, saffron, curry spices et al	Antibacterial, boost efficacy of DNA repair and detoxifying enzymes, modification of known carcinogenic compounds, linalool	prostate cancer, mouth and throat cancer, stomach cancer, liver cancer, breast, ovarian, cervical and uterine cancer.
Pulses, Beans, Whole Grains, Soya, Seeds and Fibre	Phytochemicals / phyto oestrogens Anti-oxidant, Anti-inflammatory, Zinc, vitamin D and E	Cancers of the circulatory and digestive system, (as well as associated organs), prostate and testicular cancer, breast ovarian, cervical and uterine cancer

Chapter 4:
Diet Colorectal and Breast Cancer

Approximately 1.2million new diagnoses of colorectal cancer are made globally every year, a number which represents about 10% of the total. For decades the excessive consumption of red meat and alcohol have been considered to be the primary drivers of this form of cancer. Humans are unique in that we are the only animals that develop intestinal cancers as a result of eating red meat. Which I guess if you want to be militant about it adds substance to the argument "*that we are not natural carnivores*", but that is a hot potato discussion for the local hostelry. For as long as I can remember (and I'm in my fourth decade) the link between red meat and cancer has been established but not as yet understood. In particular, the ingestion of red meat is linked to pancreatic, stomach and colorectal (bowel cancer). The latest recommendation to consume no more than 500g of red meat per week and avoid as much as possible processed meats have been given a new impetus. Overall, science has known for the association between the chemistry of red meat and the incidence of the three cancers mentioned above but no causative mechanism has hitherto been established.

Ok, the association first and then the new suggested mechanism! All red meats and many processed types of meat contain high concentrations of saturated fats and the toxicity of these fats to the human colon (amongst other impacts) are well known. However, all red meats contain the protein haemoglobin and the new research builds on earlier studies which have suggested a strong role for haemoglobin in promoting the toxicity (i.e. carcinogenesis) of these same saturated fats. Research published in the year 2000 suggests that laboratory animals fed a high fat / haemoglobin diet had a higher incidence of colonic toxicity across the board (including cancer) as compared to control and low fat /low haemoglobin eating populations of animals. In general terms, the western diet is anything up to 40% fat and so the association is simply that if you have a high fat diet and you are eating too much red meat then your risk of colono-rectal cancer is increased. Furthermore, if you are consuming more than the recommended units of alcohol and / or smoking regularly your risk of developing this form of cancer increases by up to 1/5th. In essence, the presence of haemoglobin in red and processed meats goes some way to explaining why red meat is from the perspective of cancer so much more dangerous than white meats such as poultry. The impetus alluded to above is derived from research published in late 2014.

The paper asserts that long-term ingestion of a sugar known as neu5gc could be responsible for red meat induced carcinogenesis. This particular carbohydrate is found in elevated concentrations in red meat and carnivorous animals, but not in human beings. The neu5GC molecule is not readily metabolised by homo-sapiens but is (according to the research) present in high levels in the cancerous tissue of both laboratory animals and human cancer patients. Further research from the University of California established that neu5gc is present in red meat (including mutton and lamb) as well as pork. Previous research also published in autumn 2014 established that the compound is readily transported by the circulatory system. Such findings lead to the creation of a firm bottom line which is that neu5gc is in effect a foreign substance and as such provokes an inflammatory response from the human immune system. In addition, neu5gc is readily incorporated into the cells of various human tissues and for colorectal cancer, this means the cells of the alimentary canal, principally the stomach and large intestine (colon). Clearly, further research is needed but the current hypothesis is that the long-term presence of neu5gc in the diet will (all variables considered), promote an immune response which in turn facilitates tumour formation. Aside from the alimentary canal the findings imply that the human liver could also be a site of neu5gc carcinogenesis. It must be stressed that these cancers occurred in laboratory animals which are engineered to develop certain cancers and were fed a specific diet containing very high levels of neu5gc. The researchers are also at pains to promote the nutritional benefits of red meat as part of a balanced diet. In short, they do not categorically state a causative link which is equivalent to that established to cigarette smoking. Having made such disclaimers clear, such research cannot help but give those of us who choose to eat red meat some food (literally) for thought.

The above section represents a tiny fraction of the research conducted on the role of red, processed and cured meats in the occurrence of colorectal cancer. Hence the picture is far from complete and if you are a meat eater there are ways to promote the excretion of potential carcinogens. Put simply you need to eat more fresh vegetables, as well as herbs and spices of all kinds. There is plenty of research which shows that in clinical (human) trials many of the potential carcinogens found in red meat (no matter how it is cooked) can be excreted by the compounds found in green, leafy and coloured vegetables. Whether this turns out to be the case or not if you are an omnivore you need to take this particular course of action. Not only will you reduce your risk of developing colorectal cancer (and believe me it is horrible, I've checked), but you will improve your overall health and well-being. A similar position can be stated with the intake of dietary fibre, which is simply that if you are eating more fresh fruit and vegetables, then you are eating less of the foods which compose the Western diet and that by definition has to be good. Put simply various epidemiological studies indicate that individuals who eat more plant based foods than red meat based foods have a lower risk of developing colorectal cancer. I repeat the above point and state that I am not asserting a causative link, but I do assert that the risk of developing this form of cancer is significantly reduced. I invite the reader to peruse the research (primary) and secondary (newspaper and journal) literature and show that this is not the case.

According to the WHO in 2012 over 500,000 women were killed by the onset of breast cancer. It is also along with most other cancers a disease associated with ageing. In the industrialised world, approximately 93% of all diagnoses are for women aged over 40. In the US approximately 40,000 women are predicted to die from this highly aggressive form of cancer in 2015 alone. The figures for the UK as of 2012 were approximately 11,500 fatalities, with approximately 10% of this figure residing in Scotland. Almost all of these deaths are a result of the breast cancer spreading (metastasizing) to other biological sites (organs) within the body. It is must be pointed out that breast cancer does occur in the male of our species but it is exceptionally rare. In the UK the ratio is approximately 160:1 female to male fatalities. In the global south where health care provision is lacking to the point of deliberate murder, the rate of diagnoses for women under 40 reaches approximately 20%. Breast cancer is the single biggest cause of cancer mortality in women and is the second biggest killer overall; only lung cancer is responsible for more deaths.

As indicated previously when the fibre is eaten in the form of grains and wheat bran (gluten intolerance notwithstanding) it may have a role in preventing the onset of certain cancers and this includes breast cancer. Part of this association is that if a woman is following a plant based diet she is not going to be eating the fats which are thought to promote the onset of breast cancer. Dietary roughage (fibre) could have a major impact on preventing breast cancer (in pre-menopausal women) because it has the ability to bond with oestrogen. We live in a world that is for one reason or another awash with elevated levels of oestrogen. As a class of hormones, they are implicated in many negative biological impacts of which breast cancer is but one. Overall, the intake of dietary fibre is well correlated with reduced incidences of breast cancer in pre-menopausal women, but the association is not clear for post-menopausal women. Other studies indicate a very real oestrogen removing role for the compounds contained within cruciferous vegetables, particularly for post-menopausal women. Unfortunately, in terms of ingesting these vegetables, the scientific conclusions are ambiguous. All that can be said is that such foodstuffs are undoubtedly healthy, but in terms of preventing breast cancer the jury is still deliberating. In terms of fibre metabolism, the oestrogen is filtered out of the circulatory system by the liver and it is then transported to the digestive system where it binds to chemically active sites in the fibre and / or its metabolites. Then both substances are excreted and so the thinking is that the more fibre in the diet, the more unwanted (excess) oestrogen is excreted and so the lower is the probability of developing breast cancer. However, as with most research connected with cancer no definite process has been shown to occur.

A principle reason why breast cancer is such a killer is because the breast tissue itself is exceptionally sensitive to the development of tumorous cells. In turn, there are several reasons for this sensitivity. One of the many roles of the female sex hormones (collectively termed the oestrogens) is to stimulate the division of the breast cells. The more rapidly the breast cells divide and the greater is the exposure to carcinogens than the concurrent risk of developing breast cancer will increase. This basic principle explains why cancer is so much more common in tissues such as the skin, breast, colon, lungs and the uterus, but relatively uncommon in the nervous system. In addition for women who have never been pregnant the breast cells themselves are immature as compared to breast cells that have undergone any degree of lactation. It has been known for several decades that in the long run (with all other parameters being equal) that pregnancy reduces the overall risk of developing breast cancer. This risk is further reduced if breastfeeding is maintained throughout the weaning of the infant. As of 2015 the association between pregnancy and breastfeeding is not understood. However, limited research very strongly indicates that the expression of the genes related to regulating the cell cycle and the transmission of chemical signals between immature and mature breast cells may result in a more robust defence against the onset of cancer.

It is well established that immature breast cells have a greater affinity for carcinogens than mature cells. Furthermore, immature cells are less effective at repairing or removing damaged or defective DNA than their mature counterpart. In other words, the breast tissue of younger women, as well as older and/ or menopausal women that have not had children, is more prone to cancer than that of women who have had at least one pregnancy that has come to term. The basic difference between immature and mature breast cells is that the latter are able to manufacture breast milk. Hence it is particularly important for any female person who fits this basic profile to minimise their exposure to carcinogens. Puberty is a particularly crucial time because the breast cells themselves are immature and are rapidly dividing. As with other specialist cells the breast cells contain genes that function in an integrated fashion with the oestrogen hormones along with the products of digestion to keep the breast tissue healthy. In short breast cancer occurs when these processes break down. One symptom of such a collapse of normal biology is the metastasis of breast cancer cells to the lymph nodes found underneath the female arm. In essence, the nodes are entry points to the lymphatic component of the human circulatory system. From such sites, tumorous cells are able to spread rapidly to other nodes, with a particular affinity for the bones, liver and lungs. At this juncture an additional turn presents itself. We are taught from an early age that calcium is essential for healthy bone development. More precisely it is the salts of calcium and phosphorous in conjunction with the presence of vitamin D (which helps regulate the process) that enable the growth of a healthy and functioning skeletal system. A diet rich in calcium is also implicated in reducing the occurrence of colorectal cancer and so it would seem sensible to ensure that calcium-containing foods are regularly eaten. In terms of breast cancer, it is well established (if not self-evident) that a healthy skeletal system is going to be less susceptible to penetration by cancerous cells transported from the primary tumour. Hence one can assert that a well-balanced diet could help prevent the metastasis of breast cancer, at least as far as the human support and locomotion system is concerned.

The reader can be absolutely clear that as we follow the correct dietary advice research into new treatments for breast cancer continues apace. For example, scientists at the University of Edinburgh have uncovered a mechanism by which cancerous breast cells can spread through the circulatory system (undergo metastasis) and produce secondary cancers in the lungs of laboratory mice. The researchers assert that they have effectively blocked the chemical signals which allow secondary cancers to develop in these animals. Clearly, the hope is that such developments will translate into therapies for human beings. A principle reason why breast cancer is so dangerous to the woman who has developed it is the ability of primary cancer to undergo prolific metastasis. It is known that a class of white blood cells known as macrophages are formed by the immune system in response to infection. Previously, research from the same university has shown that for breast cancer to spread the tumorous cells and the macrophages need to communicate via the cytokine chemicals mentioned in the *"diabetes book"*.

The fact that the cancerous cells and normal cells can actually *"talk to each other"* in this manner is another factor which underlies the complexity and downright uncertainty intrinsic to the current state of research. In essence, the breast cancer cells are carried by the circulatory system via the macrophages to the lungs, where the secondary tumour begins to grow. In this latest research when the signalling mechanism between the macrophages and the cancerous cells was blocked the incidence of secondary tumour formation dropped by up to 67%. In addition, even when the cancerous cells did manage to spread it was much more difficult for them to enter the lungs. It was stated in chapter three that the biological processes that cause cancer in mammals are broadly speaking the same and this research represents but one latest example of this reality being demonstrated. In essence, potential therapies such as this example represent strategies which target specific classes of molecules without the severe side effects associated with more traditional forms of cancer treatment. These and other emergent treatments target the communication between the breast cancer tumour which may eventually mean that the cancer progression if not the cancer itself can be stopped.

Chapter 5:
Curing Cancer?

In the 21st century cancer is no longer the death sentence it once was. The two biggest reasons for this development are first that in 2015 oncologists know more about the biochemistry of cancerous cells than they did in 1960. The basic reason for increased longevity across the board with a cancer diagnosis is that science now understands much more clearly the carcinogenic process. Secondly, populations, in particular, the western world are generally speaking more informed about which substances and /or lifestyle increase the risk of cancer and so act accordingly. As our knowledge improves we are increasingly analysing the biological molecules that signal and promote the growth of the abnormal cells. The basic tenet of cancer prevention and cure is that all mammalian cells share the same basic structure. This applies to whether the cell is a skin cell or a neuron and it is well established that the life cycle of all cells is controlled by the same types of molecular signals. The ethos of cancer is that healthy cells become cancerous when these networks are changed as a result of exposure to mutagenic carcinogenic substances and /or as we age.

Over the last several decade's many cancer risk factors have been identified. These factors range from those that are common knowledge such as tobacco smoking to perhaps less known and understood factors such as the genetic makeup of the person and its relationship to their environment. In a very real sense, any discussion on the "causes" of cancer is a study in risk assessment. Cancer is not an inherited disease and so research focuses on how the different tumours grow, meaning (if prevention fails) we can seek to slow their development. If the growth of cancerous tumours is not halted they will eventually destroy the organs and organ systems which enable a person to function, resulting in their death. To put it simplistically and succinctly cancer is caused by damage to DNA. Even without exposure to carcinogens such as those found in cigarette smoke, exhaust fumes, industrial effluent, pesticides and chemical pollution, errors will build up over time. The last point is the fundamental reason why cancer is still associated with old age. Reflecting our biological complexity different mistakes build up and express themselves at different rates in different people, this is, of course, another reason why cancer is not considered a single disease.

One area where mistakes are known to occur concerns the functionality of a protein known as p53. As was indicated in the SIRT FOOD book all proteins are coded for by genes, which are sections of the base pairs which make up the entire DNA molecule. The p53 protein functions by recognising defective DNA molecules and it stops it being copied during cell division. It is also one of the most important tumour suppression proteins in the human organism. P53 additionally functions by allowing the body to recognise abnormal cellular growth and promotes the appropriate immune response. If both of these processes occur as they should the growth of cancerous cells is avoided. If the genes which code for p53 are damaged by carcinogens then a mutated (oncogenic) form of p53 will be produced and the tumour suppression capability breaks down. In effect, the body no longer recognises the growth of the tumour and it will multiply. Overall, a defective p53 protein is implicated in about half of all human cancers. A further area of research concerns the action of a gene known as "*myc*", which is involved in the transcription (copying) of DNA in the opening stages of mitosis. Should the myc gene be mutated the biochemical signals which promote cellular growth is produced at accelerated rates thus promoting tumour formation. In essence, the myc gene is *"over-expressed"* and the affected cells become unresponsive to the usual factors which regulate the cell cycle. These factors control the degree of cellular differentiation (processes which determine what type of cell will be produced), their growth rate and lifespan. The degree to which the overexpression affects such factors is related to both the type of and health of the cells concerned. Thus understanding how the normal and onco-forms of the myc gene interact with the cell cycle is pivotal to understanding tumour formation. Overall the myc gene is thought to regulate the expression of some 15% of all genes and their proteins and this is believed to include p53. The human body possesses a whole raft of tumour suppressing genes and enzymes which prevent the copying of damaged or faulty DNA. In essence, we are saying that when these metabolic processes are permanently damaged (mutated by a carcinogen) tumours begin to grow, spread and take hold of the body. In other words, cancers only really develop when damage to DNA accumulates over time and is permanent.

In 2001 a portent for the future of the treatment of cancer presented itself in the form of a drug known as Glivec. The drug was approved by the US FDA for the treatment of a rare form of cancer called chronic myelogenous leukaemia (CML) In essence this form of cancer degrades the bone marrow stimulating it to over produce immature white blood cells at the expense of mature red and white blood cells. In consequence, the immune system and oxygen carrying capacity of the patient is compromised. Since 2001 Glivec has been approved for use in the treatment of gastrointestinal and other cancers as well as a treatment for strokes. Glivec is widely seen as the first *"magic bullet"* treatment for cancer because it specifically targets the proteins which allow particular tumorous cells to grow. According to the medical literature, Glivec garners what is known as a *"complete hematologic response"* (CHR) for almost all patients who are undergoing treatment for CML. Haematology is the science of studying the blood and a CHR refers to an eventuality where the white blood cell count is returned to within the normal homeostatic range. By 2006 the survival rate for this form of cancer ranged from between 90 and 98%, with a relapse rate of approximately 17% and the interest in such therapies for treating cancer is obvious. Prior to the advent of glivec the only options available to patients were first bone marrow transplants which were dangerous (often to the point of being fatal), and painful and only a maximum of 25% of patients could even consider this choice. The second option was daily injections of substances known as interferons. The interferons are a class of proteins whose precise mode of action is not understood. They function by enhancing the response of the immune system to pathogens as well as to cancerous cells. They do not directly attack the infection or cancer. In the latter case, the interferon injection enables the suppression of the genes that control the proteins responsible for the growth of cancerous cells. In CML the interferon injections not only had serious side effects but functioned only to prolong the survival of the patient. Overall, before the advent of Glivec, the survival rate for this form of cancer was 30% for a maximum five years. The bad news is that we cannot start talking about a generic cure for cancer because Glivec will probably turn out to be a unique case, at least for the foreseeable future. The reason is that CML is but one of the many known forms of cancer and is caused by a single protein defect, whereas most other cancers have a complex and inter-related mode of action. The overall aetiology (causes) of cancer covers environmental as well as genetic factors, thus there is often no single cause and therefore single treatment for the disease. In the case of CML, it was possible to focus all effort on a single abnormal protein;

45

this is not the case with other cancers, such as breast, colorectal or lung cancer.

I am no fan of the global entity known as Big Pharma. There is simply not enough space to list the crimes of this nefarious and global agency in this particular book. However, the reader can be assured that there is more than enough empirical evidence to back support this charge. This is not to understate or undermine the work of oncologists and other scientists in the field of cancer research, but to question the objectives of the oligarch known as Big Pharma. This is a profit-driven enterprise composed of a few very large pharmaceutical companies. According to the internationally respected NGO Drug Watch Over the years 2003-2012 the 11 largest drug companies made a combined net profit which exceeded $700 billion. The same construct can be demonstrated for practically every capitalist enterprise on the planet, from transport to food production (including GMOs) the story is the same, power, corruption, lies, greed, destruction and exploitation. I invite the reader to tell me that I am wrong.

So, we really are talking seriously large piles of cash and the revenue generated from the sales of cancer treatment drugs is only one (albeit a large) component of this obscene profit. In 2012 Big Pharma pocketed a whopping $100 billion revenue from the global sales of cancer treatment drugs. Overall, global sales are increasing in a compound way to the tune of 10% per year. In 2007 global sales of cancer drugs were measured at some $75 billion in turnover and in 2014 45 new cancer medications became available, if you can afford them. In 2012 in the US some $325 billion was spent on prescription drugs (not including cancer prevention drugs). Without a doubt, the pharmaceutical companies are profiting from cancer and under the capitalist system it is in their interest to keep doing so. Consider, the undoubted clinical success of Glivec outlined above. The drug cost some £18K per patient when it was first introduced, but rapidly rose to over £20K per patient. In the US the price rise was even more disgusting, increasing from an already prohibitively high $30K to over $90K.

Now, as I said above I have nothing but respect for researchers and scientists in the field as well as every health care professional in the world and that includes the hospital porters. However, I have nothing but loathing for naked corruption and profiteering, especially if it is derived from human suffering and misery. The researchers who developed Glivec clearly need to be paid and paid they were. It cost a total of $900 million to develop the drug and it appears to have worked, which is obviously welcome. What is odious to a point far beyond criminal (yes these people are criminals) is the supposition that as of 2012 Glivec has netted the Novartis drug company almost $5billion and they are still charging the astronomically huge amounts of cash indicated above. One can only wonder at the individual financial cost to the patients' concerned or essential institutions such as the NHS which must approach the procurement of such drugs in terms of cost and not human need. I cannot find an adjective which registers enough disgust at such realities. Not only that (as is the want of the whole industry) they (Novartis) are wilfully curtailing the uptake of generic substitutes, which are chemically identical but cost significantly less than the branded product.

Overall, the lack of promotion of a healthy diet to prevent the onset of cancer is shamefully lacking from the mainstream discourse concerning the subject. The potential benefits are clear and apparent and in a sane and sensible world they would be shouted from the rooftops. I abhor quackery or unfounded assertions but my research leads me to categorically assert there are plenty of active ingredients in fresh unprocessed food (plant based or not) that have utility with both cancer prevention and the health conditions these books discuss. It is outrageous that not enough is being done to make this reality clear to the population.

Chapter 6:
Concluding remarks

The above writing does not even scratch the surface of the knowledge base which exists on the subject of cancer. I have sought to impart one crucial point to the reader and that is simply that there are literally thousands (if not more) of compounds and nutrients contained within the food we eat. Some of these such as water soluble vitamins can be immediately absorbed through the digestive system and be transported through the body. Others need to be digested, assimilated or in some way altered by the digestive enzymes or other active biological molecules within specific organs before they become useful to us. (this vast topic is for a future book). It must be inculcated that cancer itself is not unique to human beings and in many ways is a fact of life across the animal kingdom, of which we are but one component. Cancer is terrifying and mysterious in equal proportion but it is an entirely natural phenomenon. The point is that the modern lifestyle, including the western diet, has exacerbated its potency and in this context, cancer can be viewed as a preventable disease. As we age we are more likely to develop one form of cancer or another and so it is absolutely correct to state that eating healthy foods will reduce the risk of developing the condition. The active compounds contained within the food we eat have been consumed for thousands of years. Yet, it is only the advent of modern medicine that has unlocked some of the secrets as to the *"how"* and *"why"* of this biochemical efficacy. It is entirely correct and proper to state that eating a plant based and balanced diet could well be proven to be a pivotal mechanism for preventing the onset of a whole host of cancers. In my view eating a well-balanced non-western diet is a definite preventative measure and should be encouraged on an individual and community basis with immediate effect. Sadly, given the types of vested interest outlined in the final chapter, I do not see such an eventuality occurring on a global basis unless we as human beings demand it from the institutions which are supposed to operate for the benefit of us all. It must be remembered that most medicines are derived from plants; aspirin is, of course, the textbook example. Taxol which is used in chemotherapy is derived from the common yew tree is another substance firmly in the grip of Big Pharma. In terms of cancer prevention, although we may not know exactly which compounds target specific cancer, we can say that eating as wide a possible range of all foods will reduce your risk of developing cancer. Hence, the more rapidly this lifestyle choice is made, the less likely it will be that you as an individual will need to have contact with the nefarious construct outlined in the final chapter and you will likely live longer.

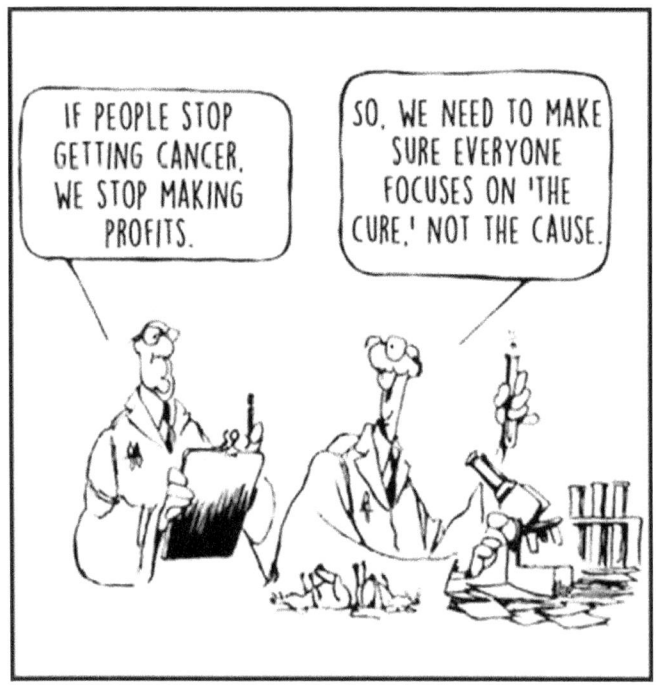

General Cancer Sources

http://www.who.int/mediacentre/factsheets/fs297/en/

http://www.who.int/mediacentre/news/releases/2003/pr27/en/

http://www.cancer.org/acs/groups/content/@epidemiologysurveilance/documents/document/acspc-027766.pdf

http://www.cancerresearchuk.org/about-cancer/cancers-in-general/treatment/cancer-drugs/imatinib

http://www.economist.com/node/18743951/print

http://www.naturalnews.com/049816_Big_Pharma_cancer_industry_medical_profits.html

http://www.nature.com/scitable/topicpage/gleevec-the-breakthrough-in-cancer-treatment-565

http://www.ncri.org.uk/wp-content/uploads/2013/11/2013-NCRI-cancer-research-spend-Uk-2002-2011.pdf

http://www.pcrm.org/health/cancer-resources/diet-cancer/nutrition/how-fiber-helps-protect-against-cancer

http://newsoffice.mit.edu/2015/link-between-inflammation-and-cancer-0115

Breast and Colorectal Cancer

http://www.cancerresearchuk.org/about-cancer/cancers-in-general/treatment/cancer-drugs/imatinib

http://www.breastcancerfund.org/clear-science/race-class-occupation-genetics-breast-cancer-risk/immigrants-migration-studies-breast-cancer-worldwide/

http://www.medscape.com/viewarticle/806573

http://www.ncbi.nlm.nih.gov/pmc/articles/PMC3709253/

http://envirocancer.cornell.edu/factsheet/general/fs5.biology.cfm

http://www.iflscience.com/health-and-medicine/possible-link-between-red-meat-consumption-and-increased-cancer-risk-identified

http://health.ucsd.edu/news/releases/Pages/2014-12-29-sugar-molecule-in-red-meat-linked-to-cancer.aspx

http://www.drweil.com/drw/u/QAA400175/Does-Milk-Cause-Cancer.html

Specific Diet and cancer Sources

http://www.webmd.com/cancer/features/seven-easy-to-find-foods-that-may-help-fight-cancer

http://www.pcrm.org/health/cancer-resources/diet-cancer/facts/meat-consumption-and-cancer-risk

http://www.ncbi.nlm.nih.gov/books/NBK92774/

http://lpi.oregonstate.edu/mic/food-beverages/cruciferous-vegetables

http://www.ncbi.nlm.nih.gov/pmc/articles/PMC2771684/

Primary Sources (Research Papers)

http://onlinelibrary.wiley.com/doi/10.1002/ijc.1409/epdf

Mangrove Forests: One of the World's Threatened Major Tropical Environments, Ivan Valiela, Jennifer L. Bowen, and Joanna K. York

http://www.nature.com/onc/journal/v27/n50/pdf/onc2008312a.pdf

Apoptotic signalling by c-MYC - B Hoffman and DA Liebermann

http://bmb.oxfordjournals.org/content/95/1/47.full.pdf+html

The molecular and cellular biology of lung cancer: identifying novel therapeutic strategies, Alison C. MacKinnon, Jens Kopatz, and Tariq Sethi

http://www.breast-cancer-research.com/content/pdf/s13058-014-0427-5.pdf

Biology of breast cancer in young women, Hatem A Azim Jr1* and Ann H Partridge2

http://bioscience.oxfordjournals.org/content/51/10/807.full.pdf+html

http://www.nature.com/bjc/journal/v102/n9/full/6605645a.html

Cancer mortality in ethnic South Asian migrants in England and Wales (1993–2003): patterns in the overall population and in first and subsequent generations

P Mangtani[1], C Maringe[2], B Rachet[2], M P Coleman[2] and I dos Santos Silva[3]

http://carcin.oxfordjournals.org/content/21/10/1909.full.pdf+html

Red meat and colon cancer: dietary haem, but not fat, has cytotoxic and hyperproliferative effects on rat colonic epithelium

http://www.bmj.com/content/343/bmj.d6617.full.pdf+html

Dietary fibre, whole grains and risk of colorectal cancer: Systematic review and dose-response meta- analysis of prospective studies

Dagfinn Aune *research associate* , Doris S M Chan *research associate* Rosa Lau *research associate* Rui Vieira *data manager* , Darren C Greenwood *senior lecturer in biostatistics* EllenKampman *professor of diet and cancer* , Teresa Norat *principal investigator*

http://ajcn.nutrition.org/content/86/2/271.long

Folate and cancer prevention: a closer look at a complex picture, Cornelia M Ulrich

Books

http://www.pcrm.org/health/cancer-resources/diet-cancer/facts/meat-consumption-and-cancer-risk

http://www.ncbi.nlm.nih.gov/books/NBK13081/

Websites of interest

http://nutritionfacts.org

http://www.naturalnews.com

http://nutritiondata.self.com

https://www.pinterest.com/coco942001/save-yourself/

https://www.pinterest.com/coco942001/clean-food-recipes/

https://viddapublishing.com

http://viddapublishing.blogspot.co.uk/

Before you go

Thank you for purchasing my book!

If you found this book interesting and enjoyed reading it, I would really appreciate a short **review on Amazon**. All of your feedback is valuable to me, as your comments and input will be taken on board to help me make this and future books even better.

I would love hearing what you have to say. Please leave me a helpful REVIEW on Amazon.

Other Books by VIDDA Publishing

THE MEDICINE ON YOUR PLATE Series

Understanding Disease, Prevention & The Importance of Plant Based Nutrition and Diet

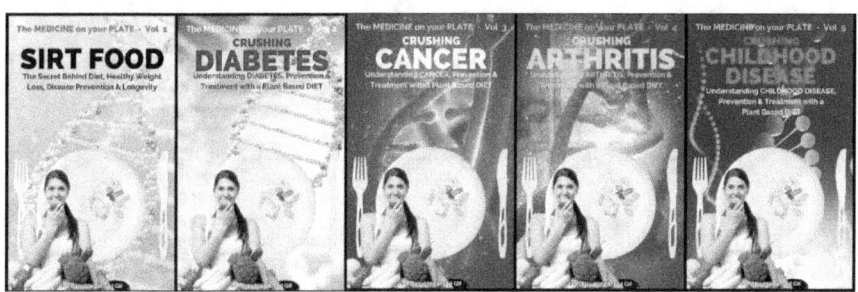

GREEN UP YOUR LIFE Series

Take control of your health and well-being by introducing Natural, Eco-Friendly habits into your daily routine.

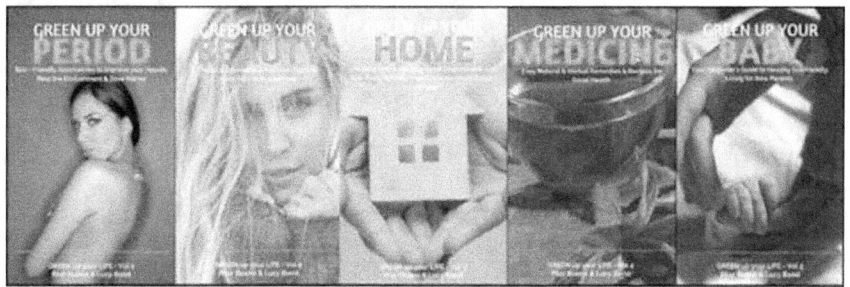

DOG TALES Series

Stories of Loyalty, Heroism & Devotion

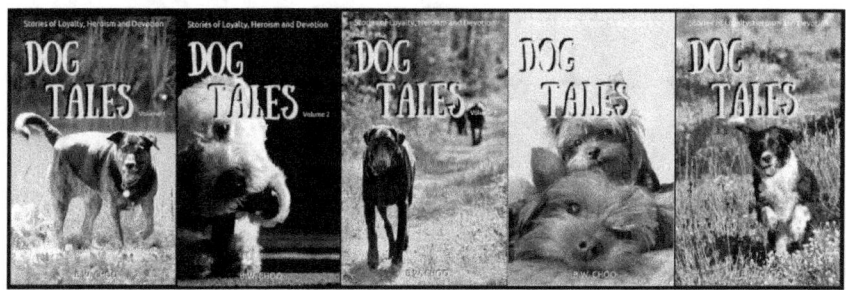

BUSINESS, INCOME & SOCIAL MEDIA Series
How to Promote, Market & Create Business with Social Media

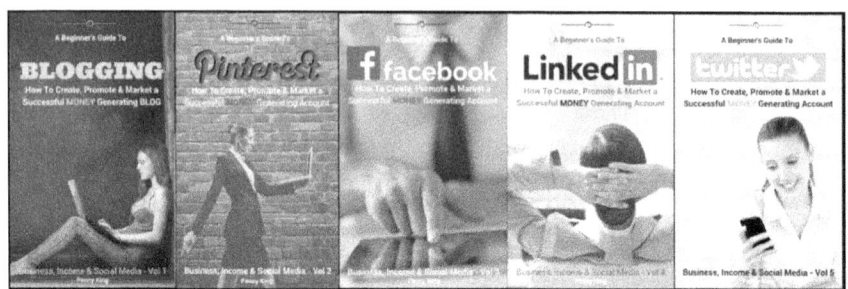

RESOLUTION TO BE HAPPY
Make yourself smile every day and banish stress and anxiety forever

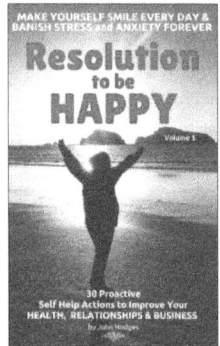

INTRODUCING GENETICALLY MODIFIED ORGANISMS - GMO
The History, Research and The TRUTH You're Not Being Told

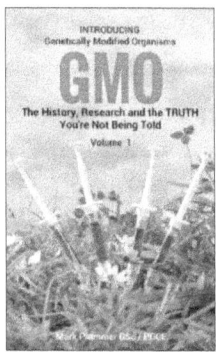

NATURAL WILD WINES

A Guide To Making Delicious Home Made Wine. Tips, Equipment, Recipes & Foraging Wild Fruits, Flowers & Herbs

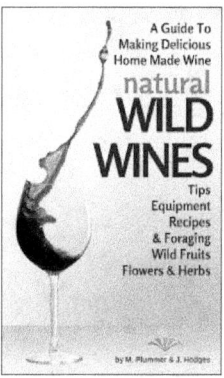

www.viddapublishing.com/books.html

Connect with John Hodges

If this book has helped you in any way or inspired you to take control of your own health and nutrition, it makes me a very happy man.

You can check out my publishing blog "Living Like You Mean It" (**viddapublishing.blogspot.co.uk**) for helpful tips, inspiration and updates on new books and free promotions coming soon.

You can also follow me on:

Twitter: twitter.com/VIDDAPublishing

John Hodges' Facebook: www.facebook.com/people/John-Hodges/550153788

VIDDA Publishing's Facebook: www.facebook.com/viddapublishing

For your Healthy, Nutritious, Green and Cruelty-Free products, equipment and gadgets, visit our online **VIDDA Health Stores** (US: **bit.ly/VIDDAstore** & UK: **bit.ly/VIDDAstoreUK**).

Also, for our favourite supplier of nutrients, sprouting seeds and health products, visit **bit.ly/BuyWholeFoodsOnline**

If you have any questions at all, please feel free to contact me at **viddapublishing.com/contact.html**

Wishing you the best of Health.

John Hodges

www.viddapublishing.com

www.themedicineonyourplate.com

www.sirtfood.com

www.greenupyourlife.org

www.ecologizatuvida.com

www.ingramcontent.com/pod-product-compliance
Lightning Source LLC
Chambersburg PA
CBHW071245280526
45788CB00004B/1585